Basic Cardiac Anatomy:

A Self-Learning Module

Gyl Garren Corona, MSN, RN,C, CCRN

Vista Publishing, Inc.

Edited by Pat Clutter, RN, M.Ed., CEN

Cover Production by Thomas Taylor of Thomcatt Graphics

Vista Publishing, Inc.
473 Broadway
Long Branch, NJ 07740
(732) 229-6500

This publication is designed for the information and education of registered nurses and interested health care professionals. The author strongly suggests that the reader seek additional educational information and resources in order to expand their own knowledge base regarding the heart. The information included in this manuscript is not to be considered the total information available on the topic.

First Edition

Printed and bound in the United States of America

ISBN: 1-880245-50-6

Library of Congress Catalog Card Number: 97-62500

USA Price $19.95
Canada Price $24.95

DEDICATION

To my family - husband Rocky, sons Rocky and Brent - for making my life special with your love and support

To my sister Joy and sister-in-law Diane - for your continual encouragement and support

To my mother Elva and mother-in-law Connie - for helping me during all of those evenings I had classes

To my nursing instructors and mentors - your guidance gave me the vision for this book

To the special women in my support group - you give more to others than you will ever realize

In memory of my father, Renton, father-in-law Rocky, and great-aunt Emilie Moore McClement ... "Set your sights on a star, and do your very best while traveling to that star"

ACKNOWLEDGMENTS

I would like to thank ...

Larry Fox for sharing his publication expertise ...

Dr. Lowell Romano for reading the draft of this manuscript and encouraging me to submit it ...

My publisher and editor for the opportunity to make this work available to members of the health care team. Your motivation and convictions inspired me throughout the editing process ...

To Betsy Toole and Cindy Radogna, Photography Services Department, St. Luke's Hospital, Bethlehem, Pa. for their artistry in taking my picture for this book.

MEET THE AUTHOR

Gyl Garren Corona has over twenty years experience in critical care nursing. Her nursing career started as a licensed practical nurse, graduating from Bethlehem Area Vocational Technical School of Practical Nursing. She credits the nursing professional demeanors and encouragement of her nursing instructors for her continuing on to her professional goal of becoming a registered nurse. She earned her associate's degree at Northampton Community College in Bethlehem, PA., BSN from Cedar Crest College, Allentown, PA, and MSN, as a critical care clinical nurse specialist, at Allentown College of Saint Francis de Sales, Center Valley, PA. Gyl has published articles in nursing journals and newsletter, and lectured on various nursing topics.

Gyl's clinical experience includes ICU, Cardiac Telemetry, Emergency Department, Nursing Administration, and Staff Development. She is currently employed as Cardiovascular Clinical Specialist at St. Luke's Hospital, Bethlehem, PA. Her professional memberships include Sigma Theta Tau, AACN, and NNSDO. Gyl is certified by AACN as a CCRN since 1985, and ANCC in Staff Development/Continuing Education since 1992. She has been named to "Who's Who in American Nursing" and "Who's Who in Young American Professionals".

Gyl lives in Leigh Valley with her family. She enjoys music, reading, crafts, and the Pocono Mountains. As a breast cancer survivor, she enjoys talking to high school girls for the "Check it Out Program". This program is designed to increase awareness of early signs and symptoms of breast cancer through breast self exam.

Table of Contents

Table of Contents

Basic Cardiac Anatomy: A Self-Learning Module

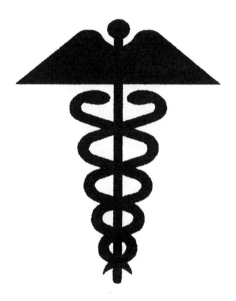

Introduction

Introduction

Upon completion of this self-learning module, the participant will be able to:

1. Discuss the 2 main functions of the heart
2. Identify the heart valves and related chambers of the heart
3. Define stroke volume, preload, and afterload
4. Discuss coronary blood flow
5. Define the Frank-Starling Law
6. Identify components of the cardiac conduction system
7. Define and compare depolarization, repolarization, and polarization
8. Compare absolute refractory and relative refractory
9. Identify the coronary arteries
10. Identify the affects of heart rate and stroke volume on cardiac output

Directions

- Proceed through this self-learning module at your own rate of speed

- Answer questions at the end of each section

- Compare your answers to the answer keys

- If you answer the questions correctly, continue to the next section

- If you have any incorrect answers, review that section again, and repeat the questions before continuing to the next section

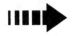

Basic Cardiac Anatomy

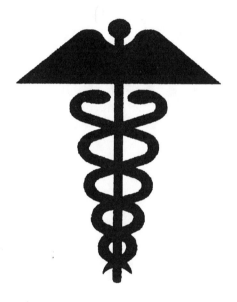

Section One

Location of the Heart

- The Heart Is Located...
  - in the mediastinum
  - with the lungs on either side
  - with the diaphragm below it...

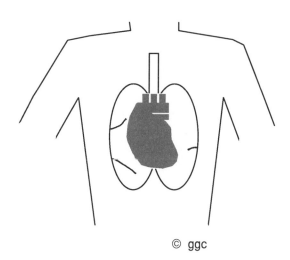

© ggc

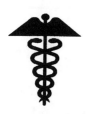

The Heart...

- The heart is slightly rotated and tilted foward, placing 2/3 of the heart left of the sternum

  with

- the apex of the heart at the 5th intercostal space, left midclavicular line (5th ICS LMCL)

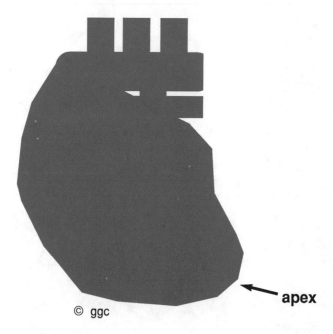

← **apex**

© ggc

REVIEW

1. What organs are on either side of the heart?

2. What is located just below the heart?

3. Where is the apex of the heart located?

ANSWERS

1. What organs are on either side of the heart?
   the lungs

2. What is located just below the heart?
   the diaphragm

3. Where is the apex of the heart located?
   the 5th intercostal space, left midclavicular line (5th ICS LMCL)

★ **ANSWER CORRECTLY?**
   NO - review previous pages
   YES - Good, continue

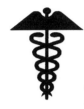

The Heart Has
2 Main Functions

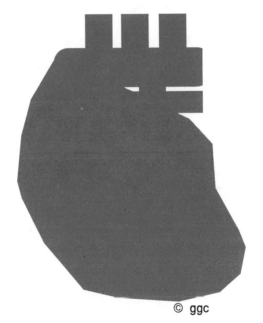

© ggc

1. To circulate blood throughout
   the body

2. To adjust the blood flow to meet
   the body's requirements...

To Circulate Blood Throughout the Body

One of the heart's main functions is to pump adequate amounts of blood to maintain perfusion to the body's organs and tissues...

- *Cardiac Output* - is the volume of blood ejected by the left ventricle into the aorta in 1 minute

- *Stroke Volume* - is the volume of blood ejected by the left ventricle with each ventricular contraction

Ventricular Systole

Ventricular Systole is when the ventricle contracts
and ejects blood

- The right ventricle ejects blood into the
  pulmonary artery to flow to the lungs

- The left ventricle ejects blood into the
  aorta to flow to the body's organs & tissues

Ventricular Diastole

Ventricular Diastole is when the ventricle is relaxed and filling with blood

- Blood flows into the ventricles from their corresponding atria...

Ventricular Diastole

During Ventricular Diastole ...

- 2/3 of the blood flow into the ventricles
  is passive, because of the pressure gradients
  in the heart

- the final 10%-30% of the blood is ejected
  into the ventricles - this is referred to as the
  atrial kick

REVIEW

Match the Following

1. ___Cardiac Output

2. ___Stroke Volume

3. ___Ventricular Diastole

4. ___Ventricular Systole

A. Volume of blood ejected with each contraction

B. Ventricular contraction

C. Volume of blood ejected each minute

D. Ventricular filling

ANSWERS

1. __C__ Cardiac Output

2. __A__ Stroke Volume

3. __D__ Ventricular Diastole

4. __B__ Ventricular Systole

A. Volume of blood ejected with each contraction

B. Ventricular contraction

C. Volume of blood ejected each minute

D. Ventricular filling

★ **ANSWER CORRECTLY?**
NO - review previous pages
YES - Good, continue

Second Function of the Heart...

Is to adjust the circulating blood flow rate
to meet the body's requirements

• **Bainbridge Reflexes**:

- *Bainbridge reflexes* increase heart rate in
response to an increase in volume of
blood returning to the atria

Baroreceptors Reflexes:

- *Baroreceptor reflexs* facilitate blood pressure and heart rate changes in response to pressure changes sensed by receptor sites in the aortic arch and carotid arteries...

  - Transmit impulses to the cardiovascular center in the medulla...

  - Stimulate sympathetic & parasympathetic nerve fibers of the autonomic nervous system...

Baroreceptors Reflexes...

With *decreased* arterial pressure...
- **sympathetic fibers** release **norepinephrine** at the nerve endings → increase in heart rate & vasoconstriction

With *increased* arterial pressure...
   parasympathetic fibers release **acetylcholine** at the nerve endings → vasodilation and vagal stimulation
- vagal stimulation → a decrease in heart rate & conduction

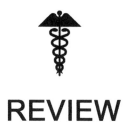

REVIEW

1. What are the 2 main functions of the heart?

2. What are the functions of the baroreceptor & bainbridge reflexes?

3. Sympathetic fibers secrete_____at the nerve endings causing <u>vasoconstriction or vasodilation.</u>
   select one answer

4. Parasympathetic fibers secrete_____at the nerve endings causing a/an <u>decrease or increase</u> in heart rate.   *select one answer*

ANSWERS

1. What are the 2 main functions of the heart?
     circulate blood & adjust blood flow

2. What are the functions of the baroreceptor &
   bainbridge reflexes?
       adjust heart rate & peripheral vascular resistance

3. Sympathetic fibers secrete *norepinephrine* at the
   nerve endings causing *vasoconstriction.*

4. Parasympathetic fibers secrete acetylcholine at the
   nerve endings causing a *decrease* in heart rate.

★ ANSWER CORRECTLY?
   NO - review previous pages
   YES - Good, continue

Basic Cardiac Anatomy

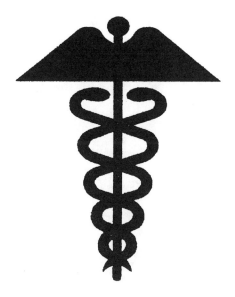

Section Two

What Can Affect Stroke Volume?

Remember- stroke volume is the amount of blood ejected with each contraction (or systole)

- *PRELOAD* - the amount (volume) of blood that fills the ventricle at the end of diastole

- *AFTERLOAD* - the resistance to ejection of blood from the ventricle

- *CONTRACTILITY* - ability of the cardiac muscle fibers to shorten and eject blood...

Cardiac Output

Remember - *Cardiac output (CO) is the volume of blood ejected from the left ventricle into systemic circulation in 1 minute*

cardiac output (CO) = stroke volume(SV) x heart rate(HR)

- **Normal CO = 4 - 8 Liters/minute**

What Can Affect Cardiac Output?

- *CHANGE IN HEART RATE -*

  - an *increase* in *heart rate* increases *CO*

  - an *increase* in *heart rate* decreases *ventricular filling time*

  - a *decrease* in ventricular filling causes
    - a drop in CO
    - an increase in myocardial oxygen demand
    - a decrease in coronary artery perfusion time

  - with a *decrease* in *heart rate*, CO usually decreases...

What Can Affect
Cardiac Output (CO)...

• *CHANGE IN STROKE VOLUME (SV) -*

   • increase in sympathetic activity ⟶ increase in

   contractility (positive inotropy) ⟶ increase

   in stroke volume ⟶ increase in CO

Change in SV (continued)...

- increase in preload

  ↓ ↓

- increase in fiber stretch

  ↓ ↓

- increase in force of contraction

  ↓ ↓

- increase in SV and CO...

Frank-Starling Law

The heart's capability to adjust to an increase in blood flow returning to the heart...

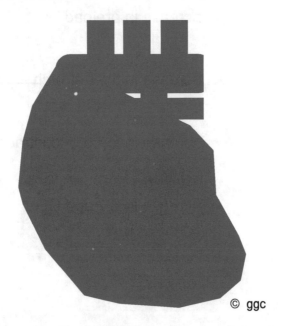

© ggc

• the further the cardiac muscle is stretched during the diastole (preload)... the more forceful the next systole (contraction)

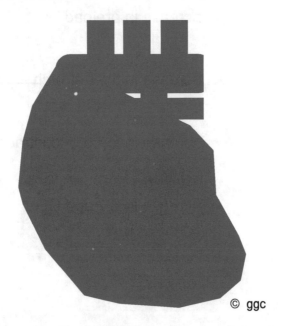

Change in SV (continued)...

• Increase in afterload ⟶ decrease in SV & CO

• Decrease in afterload ⟶ increase in SV & CO

What can Affect Cardiac Output (CO)...

CHANGE IN BLOOD VOLUME RETURNING TO THE HEART-
decrease in venous return ⟶ decrease in preload ⟶ decrease in cardiac filling, SV, & CO

increase in venous return ⟶ increase in preload ⟶ increase in cardiac filling, SV, & CO

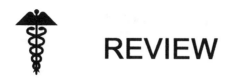 # REVIEW

Match & Answer the Following:

1. ____Preload

2. ____Afterload

3. ____Contractility

A. Resistance to ventricular ejection of blood

B. Ability of cardiac muscle fibers to shorten

C. Amount of blood in the ventricle at the end of diastole

4. What can affect cardiac output?

5. Define the Frank-Starling Law.

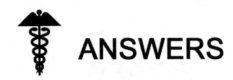

ANSWERS

Match & Answer the Following:

1. <u>C</u> Preload

2. <u>A</u> Afterload

3. <u>B</u> Contractility

A. Resistance to ventricular ejection of blood

B. Ability of cardiac muscle fibers to shorten

C. Amount of blood in the ventricle at the end of diastole

4. What can affect cardiac output?
   Changes in heart rate, stroke volume, and/or venous return to the heart

5. Define the Frank-Starling Law.
   The further the cardiac muscle is stretched during diastole, the more forceful the next contraction.

★ ANSWER CORRECTLY?
NO - review previous pages
YES - Good, continue

Basic Cardiac Anatomy

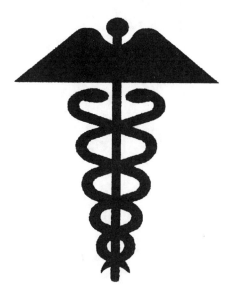

Section Three

Heart Wall Structures

1. *Pericardium* - a membranous sac that has 2 layers and provides protection against:

   a. infection from the lungs
   b. sudden over distention in heart size, and
   c. sudden impacts to the chest...

Heart Wall Structures (continued)

Pericardial Layers -
  a. *parietal pericardium* - fibrous outermost layer that supports the heart

  b. *visceral pericardium* - serous layer that covers the heart & is the inner layer of the pericardium (also called epicardium)

  c. *pericardial space* - found between the 2 layers, and has a small amount of pericardial fluid to allow the 2 layers to slide over each other without friction during contractions

Heart Wall Structures...

2. *Epicardium* - the outer layer of the heart
   - thin inner layer of the pericardium
   - coronary arteries are embedded in the epicardium

3. *Myocardium* - the middle layer of the heart
   - thickest layer
   - muscle layer - composed of muscle fibers that
     contract ⟶ pumping effect of the heart

Heart Wall Structures...

4. *Endocardium* - the inner, smooth, membranous layer that lines the chambers of the heart

5. *Papillary Muscles* - are parallel to the ventricular wall, originate in the ventricular endocardium and attach to the chordae tendineae

Heart Wall Structures...

6. *Chordae Tendineae* - tendon like attachments that prevent eversion of the tricuspid & mitral valves during systole

- attach from the papillary muscles to the valve cusps

- work with papillary muscles to open and close valves

REVIEW

1. Name the heart wall structure that protects the heart from trauma & infection.

2. What layer of the heart is home to the coronary arteries?

3. Name the muscle layer of the heart.

4. What attaches the endocardium to the tricuspid & mitral valve cusps?

ANSWERS

1. Name the heart wall structure that protects the heart from trauma & infection.
   pericardium

2. What layer of the heart is home to the coronary arteries?
   epicardium

3. Name the muscle layer of the heart.
   myocardium

4. What attaches the endocardium to the tricuspid & mitral valve cusps?
   the papillary muscles, originating in the endocardium, attach to the chordae tendineae, and the chordae tendineae attach to the valve cusps

★ ANSWER CORRECTLY?
   NO - review previous pages
   YES - Good, continue

Myocardial Cells...

Cardiac muscle differs from skeletal muscle:

- it has more mitochondria & can provide more energy for repetitive action

- it's fibers are connected to each other by intercalated discs forming a continuous network called a *functional syncytium...*

Functional Syncytium...

- *functional syncytium* - one fiber is depolarized

  and the action potential spreads along the

  syncytium to all fibers - often referred to as the

  "all or nothing" response...

Myocardial Cells...

Sarcomere - the basic functional unit of contraction

- it gives myocardial cells their striated appearance

- it is composed of fibrils

- each fibril is divided into filaments...

Filaments...

- Filaments are made of contractile proteins... there are 4 contractile proteins

  - myosin - forms thick filaments

  - actin, troponin & tropomyosin - form thin filaments

Myocardial Cells...

- *Sarcomeres* are separated from each other by

  thickened membrane *(sarcolemma)* at the end of

  each sarcomere - these are called *intercalated discs*

- *Intercalated discs* rapidly spread electrical impulses

  across the functional syncytium for cardiac contraction...

The Sarcomere...

- When cardiac cells are stimulated - calcium leaves its storage area in the *sarcoplasmic reticulum*, travels via the *T -Tubules* into the cells, resulting in contraction...

The Sarcomere...

- At the end of a contraction - free calcium is

  absorbed back into the cell's sarcoplasmic

  reticulum, traveling across the cell membrane,

  and out of the cell resulting in relaxation

REVIEW

1. What gives cardiac muscle the energy needed for repetitive contractions?

2. Name the basic functional unit of contraction.

3. _____is released from the sarcoplasmic reticulum, travels through the sarcomere, and causes a contraction.

ANSWERS

1. What gives cardiac muscle the energy needed for repetitive contractions?
   abundant mitochondria

2. Name the basic functional unit of contraction.
   the sarcomere

.3. ***Calcium*** is released from the sarcoplasmic reticulum, travels through the sarcomere, and causes a contraction.

★ ANSWER CORRECTLY?
 NO - review previous pages
 YES - Good, continue

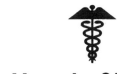

The Heart's Chambers

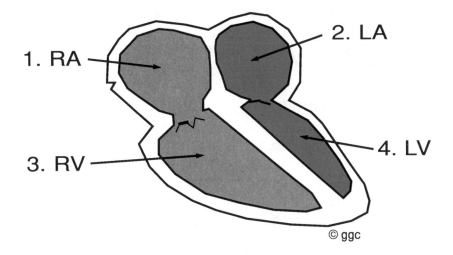

1. RA

2. LA

3. RV

4. LV

© ggc

The heart has 4 chambers

1. the right atrium (RA)
2. the left atrium (LA)
3. the right ventricle (RV)
4. the left ventricle (LV)

The Atria

- Are thin walled, low pressure chambers
- the pressure in the RA is 2-6mmHg
- the pressure in the LA is 4-12mmHg

- the RA receives systemic venous blood from the
  - (a) superior vena cava
  - (b) inferior vena cava
  - (c) coronary sinus...

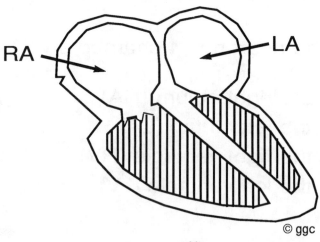

RA

LA

© ggc

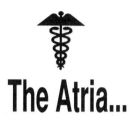

The Atria...

- the LA receives oxygenated blood from the lungs through the pulmonary veins

- the atria are reservoirs for blood flowing into their respective ventricles

- the atria are divided by the intra-atrial septum

intra-atrial septum

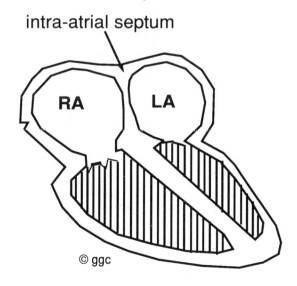

RA   LA

© ggc

The Ventricles

- The ventricles are the major "pumps" of the heart

- The muscle walls are thicker than the atria walls

- The intraventricular (IV) septum divides the RV & LV

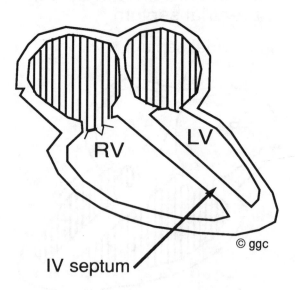

RV   LV

© ggc

IV septum

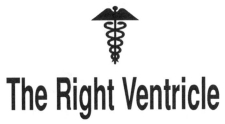

The Right Ventricle

- The right ventricle (RV) receives blood from the right atria (RA)

- The pressure in the RV is 15-30mmHg

- The RV pumps deoxygenated blood into the pulmonary circulation through the pulmonary artery (PA)

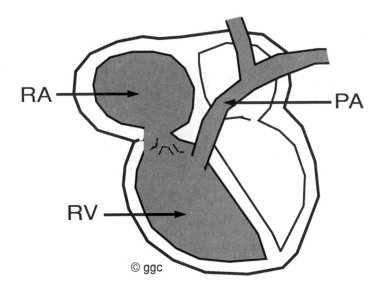

RA

PA

RV

© ggc

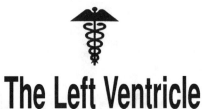

The Left Ventricle

- Has the thickest walls of the chambers

- Normal pressure is 120 mmHg systolic & 1-10 mmHg diastolic

- Is cone shaped, and contracts with a squeezing motion to overcome the high pressure (afterload) in the aorta

- Ejects blood into the aorta & systemic circulation during ventricular systole

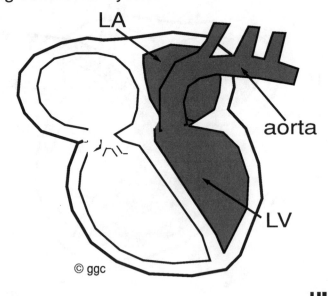

© ggc

Blood Flow From Atria to Ventricles

- approximately 70% of the blood in the atria flows passively from the atria into the ventricles

- the remaining 10-30% of the blood in the atria is forcefully ejected into the ventricles with an atrial contraction

- this forceful atrial contraction is called the *atrial kick*

REVIEW

1. Name the 4 chambers of the heart.

2. What is the main function of the atria?

3. Define the atrial kick.

4. What chamber pumps blood to the lungs?

5. What chamber pumps blood into systemic circulation?

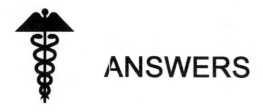 # ANSWERS

1. Name the 4 chambers of the heart.
   The right & left atria, right & left ventricle

2. What is the main function of the atria?
   The atria function as reservoirs for blood flowing into the ventricles

3. Define the atrial kick.
   The atrial kick is the atrial contraction that ejects the last 10-30% of blood into the ventricles

4. What chamber pumps blood to the lungs?
   The right ventricle

5. What chamber pumps blood into systemic circulation?
   The left ventricle

★ ANSWER CORRECTLY?
  NO - review previous pages
  YES - Good, continue

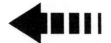 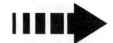

Heart Valves

- Heart valves retain blood in one chamber until the next chamber or vessel is ready to receive blood.

- Each valve responds to pressure changes
  - valves open when the pressure in the chamber filling with blood (behind the valve) is greater than the pressure in the chamber or vessel that will receive the blood...

Heart Valves

Valve response to pressure change...

► example #1- pressure in the filled RA is greater than the pressure in the RV, the tricuspid valve opens, and blood flows into the RV

► example #2- pressure in the filled RV is greater than the pressure in the PA, the pulmonary valve opens, and blood flows into the PA

Two Types of Heart Valves

1. *Atrioventricular Valves* - are located between the atria and the ventricles

   Ticuspid Valve -
   • located between the RA & RV
     (hint-think RT for right & tricuspid)

   Mitral Valve -
   • located between the LA & LV
     (hint- think L&M for left and mitral)...

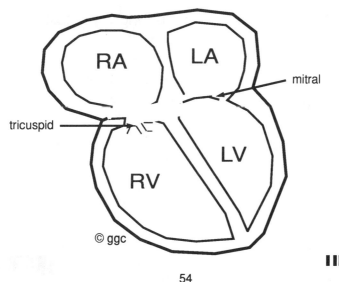

AV Heart Valves...

- allow for unidirectional blood flow into the ventricles during ventricular diastole

  - chordae tendineae attach valve cusps to papillary muscles, acting as anchors, preventing cusps from entering back into the atria at the end of a contraction

- prevent retrograde flow of blood during ventricular systole

- the first heart sound -S1, is the closure of the AV valves ("lubb")

Heart Valves...

2. *Semilunar Valves* - are located between the ventricles and their respective arteries

   Pulmonary Valve -
   • located between the right ventricle (RV) & pulmonary artery (PA)

   AorticValve -
   • located between the left ventricle (LV) & aorta

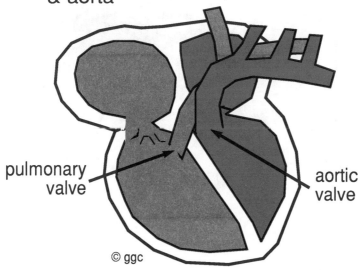

pulmonary valve

aortic valve

© ggc

Heart Valves...

2. SEMILUNAR VALVES:

- Opening occurs with contraction (ventrical systole) pressure in the ventricle is greater than the pressure in the corresponding artery

- Closing occurs with relaxation (ventricular diastole)- pressure in the artery is greater than the pressure in the ventricle.

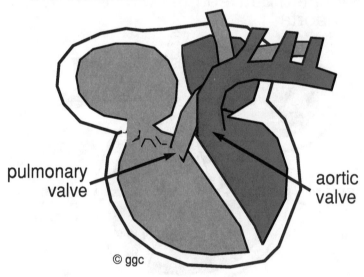

pulmonary valve

aortic valve

© ggc

Heart Valves...

SEMILUNAR VALVES...
- allow unidirectional blood flow during systole, & prevents retrograde blood flow during diastole

- the second heart sound, S2, is the closure of the semilunar valves ("dupp")

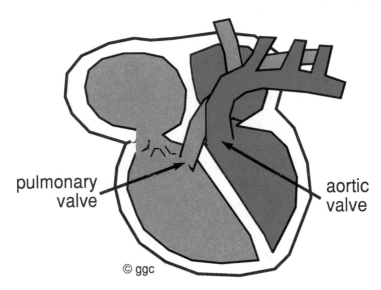

pulmonary valve

aortic valve

© ggc

REVIEW

1. Name the atrioventricular valves and their locations.

2. Name the semilunar valves and their locations.

Match the Following

3. _____ S1

4. _____ S2

A. closure of the pulmonary & aortic valves

B. closure of the mitral & tricuspid valves

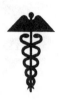

ANSWERS

1. Name the atrioventricular valves and their locations.
   - *the tricuspid valve divides the RA & RV*
   - *the mitral valve divides the LA & LV*

2. Name the semilunar valves and their locations.
   - *the pulmonary valve divides the RV & pulmonary artery*
   - *the aortic valve divides the LV & aorta*

Match the Following

3. __B__ S1

A. closure of the pulmonary & aortic valves

4. __A__ S2

B. closure of the mitral & tricuspid valves

★ ANSWER CORRECTLY?
NO - review previous pages
YES - Good, continue

Basic Cardiac Anatomy

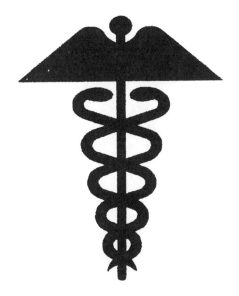

Section Four

Blood Flow Through The Heart...

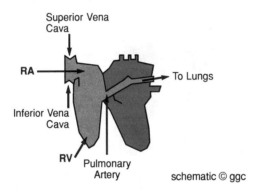

Superior Vena Cava

RA → To Lungs

Inferior Vena Cava

RV — Pulmonary Artery

schematic © ggc

→ Unoxygenated blood from the body enters the RA through the superior vena cava and inferior vena cava...

→ blood flows from the RA, through the tricuspid valve into the RV...

→ from the RV, blood flows through the pulmonary valve into the pulmonary artery (the only artery that carries unoxygenated blood) to travel to the lungs for oxygenation...

Blood Flow Through The Heart...

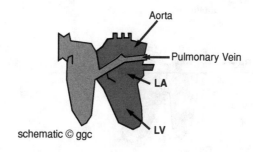

Aorta

Pulmonary Vein

LA

LV

schematic © ggc

➤ oxygenated blood from the lungs enters the LA through the pulmonary veins (the only veins that carry oxygenated blood)

➤ blood flows from the LA through the mitral valve into the LV...

➤ from the LV, blood flows through the aortic valve, into the aorta, and into systemic circulation...

Blood Flow Through The Heart...

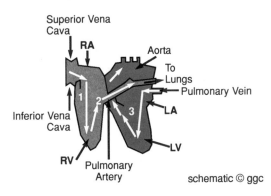

Superior Vena Cava

RA

Aorta

To Lungs

Pulmonary Vein

Inferior Vena Cava

LA

1

2

3

RV

Pulmonary Artery

LV

schematic © ggc

KEY: RA = right atrium   LA = left atrium
       RV = right ventricle   LV = left ventricle
       1 = tricuspid valve   3 = mitral valve
       2 = pulmonary valve   4 = aortic valve

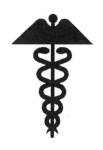

REVIEW

Identify blood flow through the heart,
naming the chambers & valves

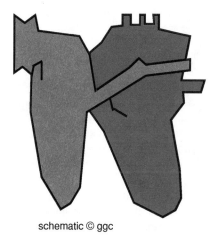

schematic © ggc

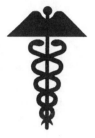

ANSWER

Identify blood flow through the heart,
naming the chambers & valves

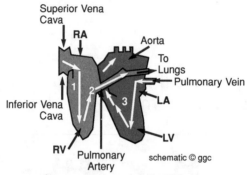

Superior Vena
Cava
RA
Aorta
To
Lungs
Pulmonary Vein
1
2
3
LA
Inferior Vena
Cava
LV
RV
Pulmonary
Artery
schematic © ggc

→ Unoxygenated blood enters the RA from the inferior vena cava &
superior vena cava
→ flows through the RA to the RV with the opening of the tricuspid valve
→ RV contracts and blood flows through the pulmonary valve into the
pulmonary artery to the lungs for oxygenation
oxygenated blood returns to the heart via the pulmonary valve into the
pulmonary artery to the lungs for oxygenation
→ oxygenated blood returns to the heart via the pulmonary veins, entering
the LA
→ blood flows from the LA to the LV with the opening of the mitral valve
→ LV contracts, ejecting blood through the aortic valve, into the aorta and
out into systemic circulation

* ANSWER CORRECTLY?
NO - review previous page
YES - Good, continue

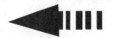 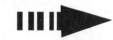

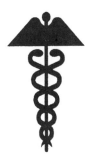

• Coronary Arteries

• Coronary arteries deliver oxygenated blood to the myocardium & conduction system

• The coronary arteries fill with blood during ventricular diastole...

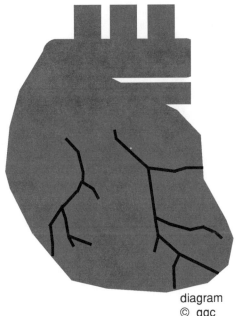

diagram
© ggc

Coronary Arteries...

- The coronary arteries branch off the aorta...
  - are embedded in the epicardium
  - circle the heart

- They branch into arterioles & capillaries...
  - supplying the myocardium & endocardium with blood...

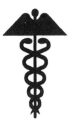

The Right Coronary Artery (RCA)

- Supplies:
    - SA node in approximately 55% of the population
    - AV node in approximately 90% of the population
    - Right atrium (RA) & right ventricle (RV)
    - Inferoposterior wall of the left ventricle (LV)...

    - 80% of the population has a posterior descending branch of the RCA
        - This is then referred to as "right dominant"

RCA ———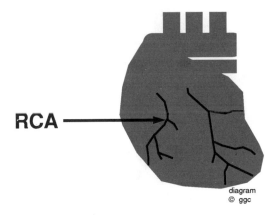

diagram
© ggc

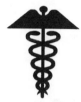

Right Coronary Artery (RCA)...

- The *Posterior Descending Branch-* found in the posterior interventricular groove...
  - Supplies blood to:
    - the right ventricle
    - the inferior wall of the left ventricle
    - the posterior portion of the IV septum

- The *Marginal Acute Branch* - found at the right lateral side of the heart to apex
  - supplies the inferior wall of the right ventricle

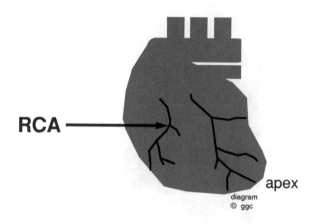

RCA

apex

diagram
© ggc

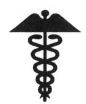

The Left Coronary Artery (LCA)...

• The LCA starts at the aorta as the *Left Main Coronary Artery* and divides into the *2 branches...*
  • *Circumflex*
  • *Left Anterior Descending* **(LAD)**

• *CIRCUMFLEX* - supplies blood to the:
  • SA node in approximately 45% of the population
  • AV node in approximately 10% of the population
  • lateral posterior wall of the LV
  • the left atrium...

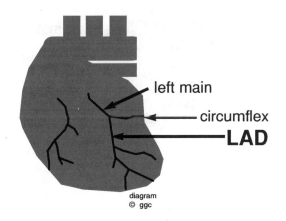

diagram
© ggc

70

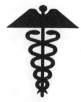

The Left Coronary Artery (LCA)...

- *Left Anterior Descending (LAD) - supplies:*
  - right bundle branch
  - the anterior wall of the LV
  - the anterior interventricular septum
  - the anterosuperior division of left bundle branch

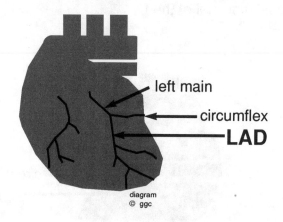

left main

circumflex

LAD

diagram
© ggc

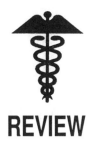

REVIEW

1. The coronary artery that supplies most of the anterior wall of the LV, and the IV septum is the
_____ coronary artery.

2. Identify the labeled areas on the diagram below

A_____

B_____

C_____

D_____

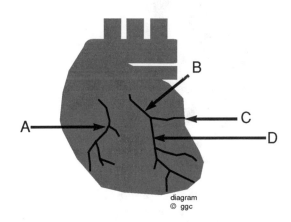

diagram
© ggc

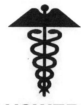

ANSWERS

1. The coronary artery that supplies most of the anterior wall of the LV, and the IV septum is the
___*left anterior descending (LAD)*___ coronary artery.

2. Identify the labeled areas on the diagram below

A. ___*right coronary artery (RCA)*___

B. ___*left Main*___

C. ___*circumflex*___

D. ___*left anterior descending (LAD)*___

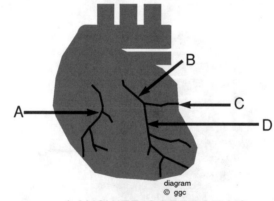

diagram
© ggc

* ANSWER CORRECTLY?
◄ ❙❙❙❙ NO- review previous pages ❙❙❙❙►
YES- Good, continue

Basic Cardiac Anatomy

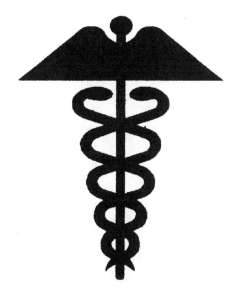

Section Five

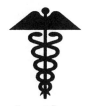

The Conduction System

The conduction system is the electrical system of the heart. It is important to understand the conduction system when interpreting cardiac rhythms.

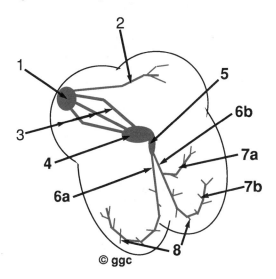

© ggc

KEY:
1. SA Node
2. Bachmann's Bundle
3. Internodal Pathways
4. AV Node
5. His Bundle

6a. Right Bundle Branch
6b. Left Bundle Branch
7a. LBB Posterior Fascicle
7b. LBB Anterior Fascicle
8. Purkinje Fibers

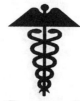

Atrial Conduction

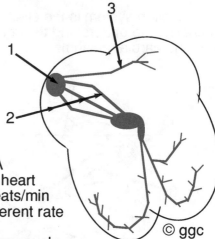

3

1

2

© ggc

1. SA Node
   • located high in the RA
   • normal pacemaker of heart
   • intrinsi rate 60-100 beats/min
   • possesses fastest inherent rate
     of depolarization
   • impulse travels simultaneously
     through the atrial walls causing immediate contraction

2. Internodal Pathways
   • transmits impulse through RA to the AV Node

3. Bachmann's Bundle
   • transmits impulse to the LA

AV Node

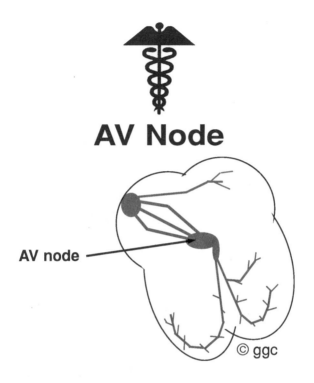

AV node

© ggc

- located at the top of the intraventricular (IV) septum

- intrinsic rate 40-60 beats/minute

- delays impulse from SA node to the ventricles to allow time for the ventricles to fill before ventricular systole

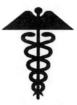

Ventricular Conduction

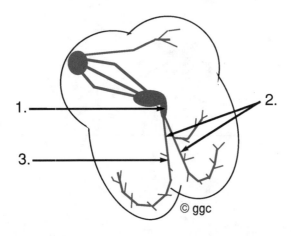

1. ⟶
2.
3. ⟶

© ggc

1. *Bundle of His* - originates at the AV node and divides into Right and Left Bundle Branches

2. *Right & Left Bundle Branches* - conduction pathways that originate at the Bundle of His

3. *Right Bundle Branch (RBB)* - conducts impulse down the right side of the IV septum through the RV

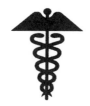

Ventricular Conduction

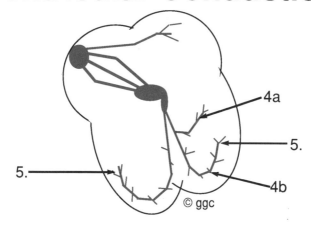

4a

5.

5.

4b

© ggc

4. *Left Bundle Branch (LBB) -* conducts impulse
through the LV, divides into 2 branches
a. anterior fascicle
b. posterior fascicle

5. *Purkinje Fibers -* terminal fibers of the conduction
system-
  • intrinsic rate 20-40 beats/minute
  • rate is slowest at the distal ends
    (2-8 beats/minute)

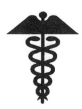

REVIEW
LABEL THE CONDUCTION SYSTEM

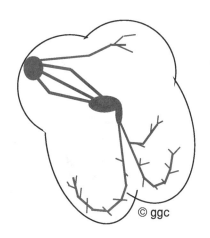

© ggc

1. SA Node
2. Bachmann's Bundle
3. Internodal Pathways
4. AV Node
5. Bundle of His

6. Right Bundle Branch
7. Left Bundle Branch
  7a. Anterior Fascicle
  7b. Posterior Fascicle
8. Purkinje Fibers

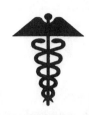

ANSWERS

LABEL THE CONDUCTION SYSTEM

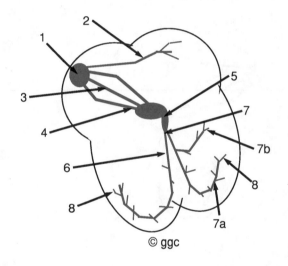

© ggc

1. SA Node
2. Bachmann's Bundle
3. Internodal Pathways
4. AV Node
5. Bundle of His

6. Right Bundle Branch
7. Left Bundle Branch
   7a. Anterior Fascicle
   7b. Posterior Fascicle
8. Purkinje Fibers

* ANSWER CORRECTLY?
NO - review previous page
YES - Good, continue

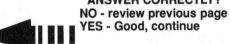
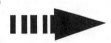

Cardiac Events During
Depolarization & Repolarization

Note: Since the LV is the "main pump", it is common to discuss the cardiac cycle from the viewpoint of the LV. Keep in mind that the same sequence of events is occurring on the right side of the heart.

Depolarization & Repolarization...

Electrical activity of the heart precedes contraction -

- *Depolarization* - "discharge" of the electrical impulse - conduction through the heart to produce a contraction (systole)

- *Repolarization* -"recovery" state - the heart is recovering from the previous depolarization & is relaxed (diastole)

- *Polarization* - "prepared" - the heart is ready for the next electrical impulse...

Electrophysiology...

- *Resting membrane potential (RMP) : -80 to -90 mV*

    - the cardiac cell is polarized, or ready for the next impulse

    - sodium ion concentration is greatest outside of cell

    - potassium ion concentration is greatest inside of cell
        - *Hint - to remember sodium is outside of the cell & potassium is inside, think of the normal serum concentrations.*
        Since serum sodium is higher than serum potassium, sodium concentration is greatest outside of the cell ...

Electrophysiology...

- *Stimulation of membrane*

  - stimulation of cell, reducing the RMP negative value is depolarization (-60 to -70 mV)

  - permeability of the cell membrane is altered

  - special channels in the membrane open permitting ion movement...

Electrophysiology

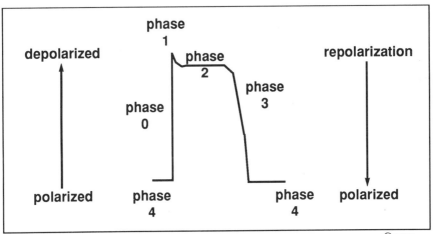

© ggc

phase 0 = depolarization -
  • sodium rapidly enters the cell

phase 1 = repolarization starts -
  • calcium slowly enters the cell
  • fast sodium channels close

phase 2 = plateau phase - continued repolarization
  • calcium & sodium slowly enter the cell
  • potassium moves out of the cell

Electrophysiology

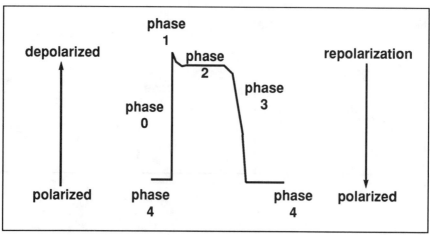

© ggc

phase 3 = rapid repolarization -
  • slow calcium channels close
  • potassium rapidly leaves cell
  • at the end of phase 3 -
       active transport system pumps potassium
       into the cell & sodium out of the cell (this causes
       the rapid repolarization)

phase 4 = polarization -
  • return to resting membrane potential (RMP)

* *Note - phases 0, 1, & 2 correspond to QRS complex
   on ECG, phase 3 with T wave, and phase 4 with the
   isoelectric line*

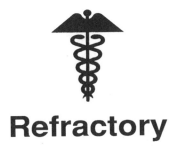

Refractory

- *Refractory* - the inability to accept or conduct an impulse

- *Absolute Refractory...*
  - phases 0, 1, 2, and the first half of phase 3

    - *absolute refractory* corresponds with the QRS and the first 1/2 of the T wave...

Absolute Refractory
QRS & 1/2 OF T WAVE

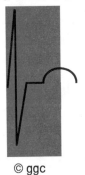

© ggc

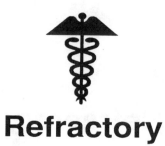

Refractory

- *Relative Refractory...*
  - during the last half of phase 3, the cell is in *relative refractory*

- *Relative Refractory* also corresponds with the last 1/2 of the T wave
     and the first 1/2 of the T wave...

Relative Refractory
last 1/2 of T wave

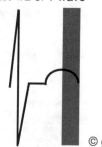

© ggc

- *Relative Refractory* is the vulnerable period of the cardiac cycle - an impulse may cause a repetitive or chaotic dysrhythmia

REVIEW

Match the Following

1. ___depolarization

2. ___repolarization

3. ___polarization

4. ___absolute refractory

5. ___relative refractory

A. unable to conduct an impulse

B. discharge & conduction of impulse

C. ready state for an impulse

D. recovery state of cell

E. a strong stimulus may cause a chaotic or repetitive rhythm

6. During depolarization,____rapidly enters the cell.

ANSWERS

Match the Following

1. **_B_** depolarization

2. **_D_** repolarization

3. **_C_** polarization

4. **_A_** absolute refractory

5. **_E_** relative refractory

A. unable to conduct an impulse

B. discharge & conduction of impulse

C. ready state for an impulse

D. recovery state of cell

E. a strong stimulus may cause a chaotic or repetitive rhythm

6. During depolarization, **_sodium_** rapidly enters the cell.

★ ANSWER CORRECTLY?
NO - review previous pages
YES - Good, continue

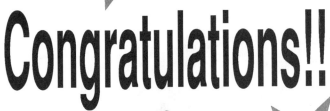

Congratulations!!

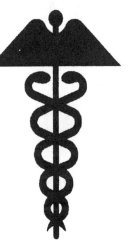

You Have Completed This
Self-Learning Module

Basic Cardiac Anatomy

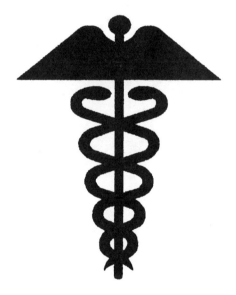

Section Six

References

Ahearns, T. (Ed.)(1991). Critical care certification preparation and review, (2nd ed.) (pp.3-53) East Norwalk, CT: Appleton & Lang.

Clochesy, J., Breu, C., Cardin, S., Whittaker, A., & Rudy, E. (1996). Critical care nursing (2nd ed.). Philadelphia: W.B. Saudners Co.

Chou, T. & Knilans, T. (1996). Electrocardiography in clinical practice: Adult and pediatric (4th ed.). Philadelphia: W.B. Saunders Co.

DeAngelis, R. (1991). The cardiovascular system. In Alspach, G. (Ed.) Core curriculum for critical care nursing. Philadelphia: W.B. Saunders Co.

McCance, K. & Huether, S. (1994). Unit IX: The cardiovascular and lymphatic systems (pp. 940-999). In Pathophysiology: The biologic basis for disease in adults and children (2nd ed.). St. Louis: Mosby

Noone, J. (1992). Arrhythmia interpretation a workbook for nurses. Springhouse, PA: Springhouse.

Woods, S., Froelicher, E., Halpenny,C., & Motzer, S. (1995). Cardiac nursing (3rd. ed.). Philadelphia: J.B. Lippincott Co.

Wright, J. & Shelton, B. (1993). Desk reference for critical care nursing. (pp.467-598). Boston: Jones and Bartlett Publishers

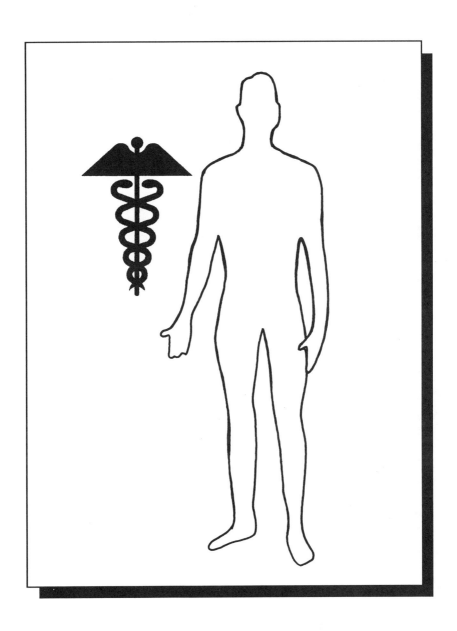